30 Day Paleo Challenge

The 30 Day Paleo Diet to Lose Weight and Live a Healthier Lifestyle.

S0-ABA-968

Sarah Stewart

Table of Contents

Introduction: Let's Go Paleo!

When you hear about something called a "paleo diet" you may be tempted to raise a skeptical eyebrow and assume that this diet with its unusual name is just another ill conceived weight loss scheme. But the paleo diet isn't some gimmick or fad; it is simply a return to the natural diet that nature intended. Harkening back to the days of our hunter gatherer ancestors in the Paleolithic Era, the paleo diet espouses the consumption of simple dietary staples such as seeds, nuts, and berries, as well as an ample supply of fresh meat.

Similar to the Atkins diet, the paleo diet cuts out a tremendous amount of carbs, but unlike the Atkins diet which just focuses on the quantity of the carbs you can cut, the paleo diet focuses on the quality of your overall health. While Atkins dieters are encouraged to gorge themselves on meat of all kinds no matter how many hormones and antibiotics are used, the paleo diet calls for you to only choose healthy meat that has been grass fed and kept hormone free.

It is no small coincidence that many Atkins dieters have suffered from heart attacks, due to their diet. Because despite their trim appearance, the Adkins recommendation to gorge on fatty meats such as bacon soaked in grease have left many with clogged arteries in their underweight bodies! Recent studies concur with this phenomenon, and have shown that the Atkins diet can increase our cholesterol and has been known to contribute to heart disease.

The paleo diet however, avoids these pitfalls because the focus of paleo is not simply the reduction of carbs but also the refinement of the actual nutrients that we put into our body. Because even if you eat low fat, low carb foods, if the nutrient value is not in sync with what your body needs, we are not going to be healthy. Like every other living organism on this planet, our bodies, and what our bodies need, have been finely tuned and designed by the external pressures of our environment.

Just like it does for any other creature on the Earth; this planet we call home, creates highly specialized nutrients that our bodies have come to depend upon in order to be healthy. And our ancestors of the Paleolithic Age would hunt and gather these resources on a daily basis. In fact they lived about 150,000 years prior to any modern convenience and yet they could extract whatever they needed from the environment without any problem.

The paleo diet seeks to reestablish those optimal nutrition conditions, and in doing this it cuts out any food that can not be obtained naturally from the environment. This means not eating anything that has been manipulated and processed after the fact. This means cutting back on grains, dairy and other processed foods and then increasing our intake of naturally occurring food items such as grass fed meat, fresh fish, eggs, plenty of vegetables, fruits, nuts and seeds. So let's go natural, and let's go Paleo!

Chapter 1: Starting Your Paleo Diet Plan

Just like anything else in this world, you have to have a game plan when it comes to getting started on your paleo diet. There are certain ground rules that you should be following from the very beginning. In this chapter we are going to explore some of the most important of those rules that you will need to follow in order to successfully reach the end of your 30 Day Paleo Challenge.

Empty Out Your Pantry And Go Shopping

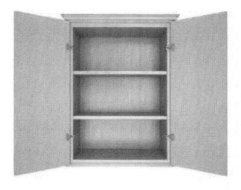

Before you do anything else, when you are starting out on a paleo diet, the first thing on your list; should be a _shopping list._ In order to be successful with your 30 day Paleo Challenge there are several food staples and ingredients that you should stock up on. But just prior to buying these items you should probably throw anything that is decidedly _un-paleo_ out of your pantry.

You can start off by just ditching anything that's loaded with sugar, wheat, or salt. If any of the food products in your pantry contains an overabundance of any of these elements, you need to consider removing them. The next thing you should get rid of, are any food items that have been created with processed grains. Get rid of cereal, taco shells, corn meal, corn flakes, corn chips (you see a pattern?), pretty much anything with corn in it! Also get rid of any items with rye, oats (oatmeal), crackers, granola or barley.

Having your fridge loaded with food that deviates from your diet plan is just going to cause you trouble later on. So if you can, try to empty out as much non-paleo food as you can. Even give it away to your friends if you have to, just try to make sure that you don't mix these non-paleo food items up with what you will actually be eating during the course of your 30 Day Paleo Challenge. After you have done this you can then work towards purchasing the actual food that you will be consuming during your 30 Day Paleo Challenge.

You don't have to be completely systematic with this, just as long as it fits in the basic parameters of a paleo centric lifestyle. This might mean going straight to the butcher of your grocery store and getting fresh, grass fed beef, chicken, goat, pork, and lamb. It would also be a good idea to stock up on fresh fish such as bass, halibut, flounder, salmon, sardines, and of course, plenty of protein rich tuna.

With your meats in order you should then move on to the fresh fruit aisle and grab up some fruit. Just be sure to put a cap on high sugar fruits such as bananas, mangoes, and watermelon. Otherwise feel free to splurge. Next on your list should be an ample amount of veggies, with the only limitation being on potatoes and legumes. Starchy veggies such as potatoes, and legumes such as lentils, peas, chickpeas soybeans, and peanuts are not included in a paleo diet and should be avoided.

People are often surprised to find out that peanuts are actually a legume and not really a part of the nut family at all. But yes, peanuts are indeed legumes, like beans, they come from a plant with pods, and they should be avoided. As for the actual nuts that you should eat, you should stock up on classic nut staples such as cashews, almonds, pecans, pistachios, and macadamia nuts.

With your nuts in order (I know that sounds kind of funny, but just bear with me here!) you should then move on to your seed supply, buying seed staples such as sunflower, pumpkin, sesame and flaxseed. Keep these seed varieties fresh in your mind, because many of them will translate into important oils that will become an integral part of how you cook and prepare your food during your 30 Day Paleo Challenge

Certain oils can be of great use in a paleo diet as cooking aids; oils such as flaxseed oil, sesame oil, olive oil, avocado oil, coconut oil, and walnut oil can be used in paleo food preparation. When starting the paleo diet you should make sure that all of these great staples of the Paleolithic Era are on your shopping list! Write them down or make a mental note, just make sure you know what foods can make the paleo diet a success when you go shopping! Because your 30 Day Paleo Challenge will be so much easier when you do!

Plan Out Your Meals in Advance

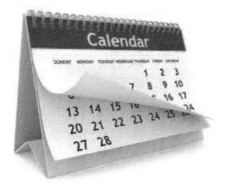

Nothing has to be set 100% in stone, but you should have a general idea of what you are going to eat and make sure that it fits within the framework of your paleo diet. Plan out what your typical morning breakfast will be; what you will have for dinner, and even your deserts well ahead of time. In doing this, make sure that you have all of the ingredients and cooking utensils you need so you won't be scrambling to the grocery store at the last minute.

Dieting is hard enough without having to struggle to put your meals together. This is precisely why diet programs like Jenny Craig are so successful, because they do that part of the work for you, and create balanced meals for you to eat ahead of time. But guess what folks? You don't need Jenny Craig to arrange your paleo diet! With a simple scheduled routine you can do it yourself!

The easiest way to keep track of your meal plan is to simply put a calendar up on your refrigerator and under each day mark exactly what it is you would like to eat in the mornings and evenings on that particular date. List clearly in each box of the calendar, "BREAKFAST, SNACK, LUNCH, and DINNER". Under each one of these headings mark down what you would like to eat for your meal during that time of day. With everything arranged ahead of time, you can eliminate confusion and mistakes. Just plan your meals in advance and you wont have to wonder about it later on.

Maintain Your Vigilance At Restaurants

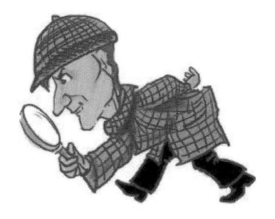

Since most restaurants are simply not paleo friendly—to say the least—the best option during your 30 Day Paleo Challenge, would be to avoid them all together. But since we can't always cook from home, and we can't always ditch outside dinner engagements with friends, family, and coworkers, we have to know how to safely navigate through what we might find in outside eating establishments.

Salads for example, should be safe on the paleo diet since most basic salads consist of roughage, and other greens that would have been compatible with the Paleolithic lifestyle of our hunter gatherer ancestors. Just avoid salad dressing like the plague, ditch croutons, and any other extra frills on your plate. Feel free to ask questions about the menu, no one will think lesser of you for it, and simply explain to your waiter or waitress, before you take your order that you are on a special diet.

Most restaurants should be understanding and at least make an attempt to accommodate you. If you tell them for example, that you would prefer your food to be cooked in olive oil rather than some of the more fattening standards that most restaurants use, they should be quick to oblige your request. You just have to ask, as long as your request isn't too elaborate and crazy; most establishments, who wish to keep their customers, will seek a way to make you happy. Just find something basic that doesn't completely break your diet and you should be fine.

Chapter 2: The Paleo Bed and Breakfast

Breakfast is the most important meal of the day, and as the recipes carefully chosen for this chapter demonstrate, a well crafted meal—paleo or otherwise—can really jumpstart your day. Mark some of these recipes down on your daily planner and your 30 Day Paleo Challenge will be a whole lot easier. The breakfast routine of our early ancestors was finely honed over a couple million years. They ate what they ate because it worked for them.

Most of us today are stuck in a routine of high carb meals that are heavy in grains such as cereal. I know that folks like their rice crispies and corn flakes, but no matter how much these cereals are touted as "healthy" that morning stockpile of grains that people shovel in their mouths—in the long run—are not good for them. We have to change our thinking all together and cut out grains completely from our diet in order to get back the health and vitality of our ancestors.

Most wouldn't think of eating fish and chicken for breakfast, but that's what our Paleolithic forefathers did and they turned out just fine! In order to finely tune your body for the rigors of the 30 Day Paleo Challenge you need to eat a breakfast that is high in protein and low on poor quality carbs, and inflammation causing grain.

If you still long for that more traditional breakfast of eggs and bacon however, don't worry! Eggs are a great part of any diet, and shouldn't be omitted, and grass fed pork prepared properly shouldn't be a problem either. In that sense, the classic standard of bacon and eggs are not really that far off the paleo menu. So go ahead and have your paleo bed and breakfast.

Paleo Baked Muffins

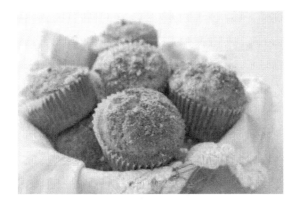

I know that for many dieters anything associated with muffins (or perhaps muffin tops) are readily avoided. But these muffins are specially made for the paleo diet and do not contain any ingredient that you have to worry about. The almond flour that they are made with make them very nutritious and they also happen to taste great! So go ahead and eat up!

Here are the exact ingredients:

1 cup of almond flour

1 teaspoon of baking powder

¼ teaspoon of salt

¼ cup of butter

½ a cup of water

3 eggs

To get started put your oven temperature at 345 degrees ad grease the cups of a muffin tin with either coconut oil, or some other kind of low fat cooking spray. Put this muffin tin to the side and get out a mixing bowl. Inside this bowl add your cup of almond flour, your teaspoon of baking powder, ¼ cup of butter, 3 eggs,, ½ cup of water and ¼ teaspoon of salt.

Mix these ingredients together well. After they've become nicely mixed, dump the mix into the cups of the greased muffin tin you had just set to the side, and place the muffin tin in the oven. Your paleo baked muffins should be thoroughly cooked after just about 10 minutes or so. A couple of these muffins in the morning is a healthy and refreshing way to start your day!

Coconut Flour Waffles

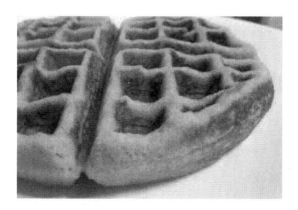

Ok, so the caveman probably didn't have a waffle iron but that doesn't mean this breakfast item is not paleo diet compatible. This recipe utilizes only strictly paleo ingredients, with the healthy staple of coconut flour as its main component. Just put these bad boys in a waffle iron and you will have yourself the best Paleolithic inspired waffles you could ever come by!

Here are the main ingredients:

1 cup of coconut flour

3 eggs

½ teaspoon of baking soda

½ cup of honey

½ cup vanilla extract

½ teaspoon salt

To get started, take out that old waffle iron that you have been hiding, plug it in and get it warmed up. While your equipment gets warmed up go ahead and get out a mixing bowl add your 3 eggs, ½ teaspoon of baking soda, ½ cup of honey, 2 cup of vanilla extract. Once these ingredients are mixed add in your cup of coconut flour, and stir it into the ingredients of the mixing bowl until it is all thoroughly mixed together. This mixture will constitute your batter.

After your batter is established, go to your waffle iron and spray it well with a good fat free, paleo friendly, coconut cooking spray so that your batter doesn't stick to the waffle iron. Once this preparation has been made you should then get out a medium sized spoon and begin to scoop up your batter into your waffle iron. Close your iron and let your waffle cook until it is nice and brown. This is a paleo bed and breakfast so good that even the crankiest of cavemen will get out of bed for it!

The Paleo Omelet

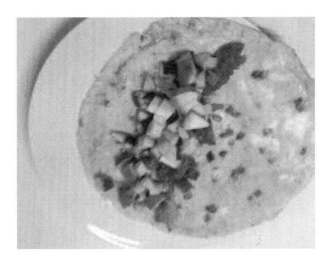

You don't have to eat pterodactyl eggs in order satisfy your paleo cravings, because this dish from the Neolithic will really make your day! It satisfies the classic bacon and egg cravings yet the healthy coconut oil this dish is cooked with won't wreck your diet. Many aspects of what makes paleo—well, paleo—is in preparation. And the Paleo Omelet is a shining testament to that fact.

Here are the exact ingredients:

2 eggs

2 strips of diced bacon

½ pound of diced mushrooms

¼ cup of coconut oil

Take a medium sauce pan and put it over low heat. Now dump in your diced bacon with your coconut oil and begin marinating the meat in your pan. After you have done this, add your diced mushrooms and then stir the whole mixture together for a minute or so. Next add your 2 eggs and stir the eggs in as well. Continue stirring the mixture until everything is thoroughly blended together into one big circle of ingredients. Now let this cook for another minute or so until the eggs solidify and bond with the other ingredients, making for one tasty paleo omelet!

Sautéed Paleo Squash and Zucchini

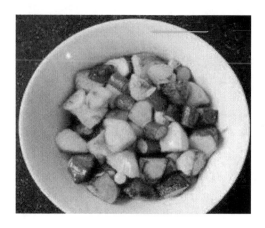

I love a good dish of sautéed veggies in the morning and this special blend of sautéed squash and zucchini doesn't disappoint. This recipe is easy to prepare and makes for a great breakfast!

Here are the exact ingredients:

2 tablespoons of coconut oil (gotta love coconut oil!)

1 finely diced onion

1 clove of minced garlic

1 chopped zucchini

2 chopped squash

½ a can of tomato sauce

First, take out a medium sized skillet and coat its insides with your 2 table spoons of coconut oil and let it simmer over high heat for about 2 minutes. Next, dump your chopped onion, squash, and garlic into your skillet. Let these ingredients cook in the pan until they are nice and crispy, before adding your garlic, and tomato sauce. Stir these final ingredients together well and then turn your burner off, letting your veggies absorb the residual heat for a few moments. This morning rush of sautéed paleo squash couldn't be easier and it couldn't taste better!

Pine Nut Scrambled Eggs

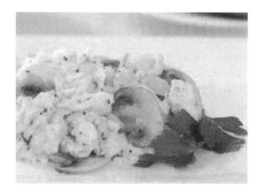

This is a tasty blend of hunter gatherer style pine nuts mixed with mushrooms and scrambled eggs! All food that could have easily been foraged by our Paleolithic forefathers! This recipe provides a satisfying blend of nuts, chives, mushrooms and eggs. The taste and texture are absolutely fantastic. As soon as you take a bite and hear that pine nut crunch you know that you are in for a treat!

Here are the exact ingredients:

2 eggs

1 tablespoon chopped chives

½ up of diced mushrooms

½ tablespoon coconut oil

½ tablespoon pine nuts

As usual with these kinds of recipes, begin the task by coating your frying pan with coconut oil over high heat. While your oil warm up, go ahead and break your eggs open and empty their contents into the pan. After you have done this, dump in your diced mushrooms, your ½ tablespoon of pine nuts, and your tablespoon of chopped chives. Your Pine Nut Scrambled Eggs are now ready for business!

The Stone Age Burrito

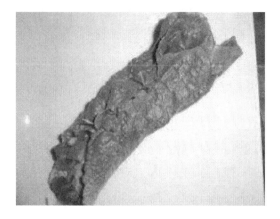

I'll let you guys in on a little secret; I love burritos. The only problem is, the typical burrito is loaded with all kinds of processed additives that can really wreck the paleo (not to mention any) diet! But this Stone Age Burrito solves that problem! Instead of using a tortilla shell, this recipe uses crisp, fresh lettuce as the wrapping material for your ingredients, providing you with a true Paleolithic gem at the breakfast table. If you ever see a caveman sitting on a rock somewhere munching on a snazzy breakfast burrito, you know where he got the idea from! (Sorry! I couldn't resist that shameless bit of self advertising!) And if its good for the caveman, it's good for you to! Try out this fantastic recipe!

Here are the exact ingredients:

¼ cup of olive oil

1 cup of chopped onions

¼ cup of chopped garlic

½ cup of chopped red bell pepper

¼ cup of ground cumin

¼ cup of cayenne pepper

½ cup chopped lean chicken

¼ cup of black pepper

2 large romaine lettuce leaves

2 eggs

Add your ¼ cup of olive oil to your pan and set your burner to its medium heat setting. Next add your cup of chopped onions to the pan and stir them into the chicken as you cook them for 3 to 5 minutes. After you have done this add in your chopped bell pepper, cayenne pepper, and ground cumin, vigorously stirring the entire contents of the pan for another few minutes.

Finally crack your eggs open into a mixing bowl and vigorously whisk them together until they consist of one fine egg paste. Dump this egg mixture into your pan and cook the eggs into the rest of the ingredients. Now just add your ¼ cup of black pepper, evenly sprinkling it over the surface of the ingredients. Put your lettuce leaves on a large plate and with a wooden spoon scoop the burrito ingredients inside your pan onto each leave of lettuce and wrap them tightly together. Your Stone Age Burritos are ready to roll!

Chicken and Veggie Breakfast

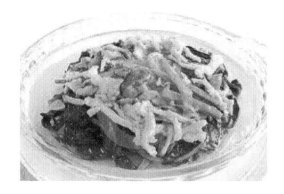

This dish is good for anyone who likes their chicken and veggies! This is a bit of a departure from the traditional breakfast, but if you feel like you need a break from eggs and bacon, this one is a good one for you! Using only the best lean chicken meat, along with a delectable blend of veggies, this breakfast dish will make you happy you woke up in the morning!

Here are the exact ingredients:

¼ cup of olive oil

½ cup of chopped onion

½ cup of chopped garlic

¼ cup of chopped asparagus

1 cup of chopped carrots

½ cup of shredded chicken

¼ cup of fresh, chopped spinach

Put a medium pan over a burner set to high heat. Place chopped onions, and chopped garlic into the pan and periodically stir the ingredients as they cook. Now add your chopped asparagus and carrots to the pan and stir them as they cook for a few more minute as well. Next, add your ½ cup of shredded chicken to the pan and let it cook for a couple of minutes as well. Turn off your burner, and add your fresh, chopped spinach, letting it cook from the residual steam that forms. Once you have done this, place a cover on the pan and drip your lemon juice onto the ingredients. This chicken and veggie breakfast is ready to enjoy.

Early Morning Salmon

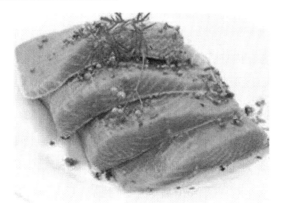

This one isn't on your typical breakfast menu but it is a Paleolithic treat all the same! Tasty fresh fish coupled with tasty mushrooms, tomatoes, and a classy blend of herbs and spices, this recipe is not to be missed! Try it out at least once during your 30 Day Paleo Challenge!

Here are the exact ingredients:

3 Salmon Fillet

¼ cup of olive oil

¼ cup of chopped fresh dill

¼ cup of paprika

¼ cup of ground black pepper

½ cup of white mushrooms

1 cup of diced tomatoes

In a medium saucepan, place a steamer basket and add 1 inch of water to the pan. Let this come to a boil, reduce your heat to just a simmer and then put your fish in the steamer and let it cook for about 20 minutes or until the fish starts to brown. After you have done this, take out a separate pan and put in your olive oil.

Next, add your ¼ cup of chopped fresh dill, your ¼ cup of paprika, and your ½ cup of mushrooms. Stir fry this mixture for a few minutes before adding in your tomatoes. Stir for another few minutes and then remove the pan from the heat altogether, and turn your burner off. As soon as your fish are done cooking, remove them as well and add your mushroom and tomato mix on top of your fish. Get up early for this morning salmon treat!

Paleo Power Breakfast

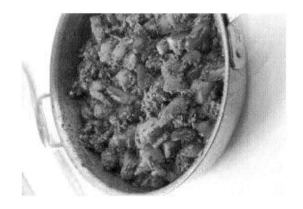

If you are especially active throughout the day, this high protein breakfast will give you the energy you need for your busy morning routine! Cooked in rich olive oil, fresh chopped turkey is roasted and marinated in tomatoes, onions and basil! Just add a couple of eggs and you've got yourself a real Paleolithic power broker! Give this recipe a chance and your wont regret it!

Here are the exact ingredients:

¼ cup of olive oil

1 cup of chopped turkey breast (already cooked)

½ cup diced tomato

½ cup diced onions

¼ cup dried basil

2 eggs

Put your frying pan over a burner set to medium heat. Now take out a small plastic bowl, add your eggs, and whisk them into oblivion! Stir these eggs as well as you can until they consist of one fine egg paste. Now pour these eggs into your pan and let them cook on medium heat for bout 1 and a half minute, as you periodically lift up the edges with a plastic utensil (spoon or spatula) just to make sure that the egg mixture doesn't stick to the pan.

Next, add your onions, tomatoes, and turkey breast. Fold your egg over these ingredients so that the cooked egg covers them like a crepe (or taco). Let the entire entrée cook like this for about 3 more minutes. Now all you have to do is cut the combination in half and put the pieces onto a large plate. All of these recipes are great for breakfast or any other time!

Chapter 3: Midday Paleo Meals

The middle of the day is when most of us get I trouble. We take one wrong detour during our lunch break at work and our whole diet is ruined. But it doesn't have to be that way. With a straightforward plan on how to tackle the midday munchies you can stay on track. In this chapter you will find some of the best possible recipes for your midday routine.

Roasted Asparagus

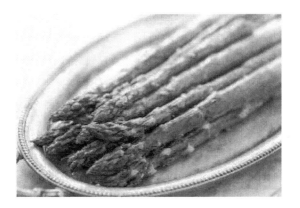

It is healthy and filling and its something that your Paleolithic ancestors would have loved to have had back in the day. As it turns out, a well roasted batch of asparagus is a hunter gatherer's treat. Depending on the climate and environment that an ancient hunter gatherer may have lived, fresh asparagus may not have been forthcoming however. But thanks to an over abundance at the local health food store, you can be sure to reap the benefit, and make a great midday paleo meal out of it!

Here are the exact ingredients:

About 15 spears of asparagus

2 tablespoons of dried out thyme

1 tablespoon of olive oil

To get started set your oven to 400 degrees, before taking out your asparagus, culling the tough ends of the veggie and placing them in the oven on a baking sheet. Liberally drip your tablespoon of olive oil and your 2 tablespoons of thyme over the asparagus. Let your asparagus bake for about 20 minutes. This is one of the simplest Paleo recipes you will ever find.

Turkey Lettuce Wrap Tacos

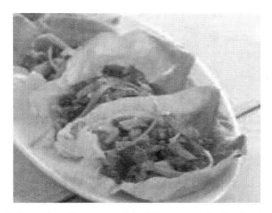

You might miss the crunch of those carbohydrate filled tacos, but this recipe calls upon a paleo transformation that cuts out the carb filled shell completely in favor for a crunchy shell made of lettuce! These turkey lettuce raps are loaded with meat, even while stocking up on plenty of tasty veggies, herbs and spices. So forget all about stopping at Taco Bell after work! Just go home and make yourself some paleo friendly Turkey Lettuce Wrap Tacos! You are going to love it!

Here are the exact ingredients:

1 teaspoon of olive oil

1 teaspoon of fresh, minced garlic

1 cup of diced jalapeno's (For that extra kick!"

1 teaspoon of cumin

¼ teaspoon cayenne pepper

2 pounds ground turkey

½ a teaspoon of salt

1 cup of diced green onions

1 cup of freshly chopped cilantro

1 teaspoon of lime juice

2 heads of romaine lettuce

Pour your olive oil into your frying pan and set your burner to high. Next, go ahead and toss in your minced garlic, and add your diced jalapenos and let the contents of the pan cook for a couple of minutes. You can then add in your teaspoons of cumin, cayenne pepper, and allow them to cook together for another minute or so. After this, add in your 2 pounds of turkey, salting with you ½ teaspoon of salt, letting the turkey cook until it turns brown.

While your turkey is browning, get out your cutting board and use it to dice up your green onions. Set these onions to the side for the moment and pickup your fresh cilantro, wash it, and then chop it into small pieces. Now stir in your cilantro with the rest of the ingredients. Now take your romaine lettuce head and cut out the core. Get rid of the rougher outer layers, before extracting the fresh lettuce underneath.

Try to peel large swaths of lettuce off of the lettuce head intact, so that you can use it hold your taco ingredients. Just take a spoon and scoop up your turkey mixture right into the lettuce and fold it into the shape of a taco! Your delicious Turkey Lettuce Wrap Tacos are now ready for their midday meal debut!

Shredded Chicken Breasts with freshly chopped Thyme

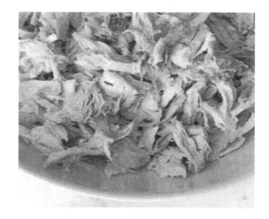

Its healthy, its delicious, and its paleo! There is noting in this recipe that our hunter gatherer ancestors couldn't have grabbed up in the wilderness. It consists of fresh chicken, with fennel seeds, mint, and a bit of thyme. Shredded chicken breasts, with just a dash of freshly chopped thyme will make just about anyone happy! This dish will make your midday meal something to look forward to!

Here are the exact ingredients:

1 lean chicken breast

¼ cup of fennel seeds

3 tablespoons of finely chopped thyme

5 tablespoons of olive oil

¼ cup of roughly torn mint

1 lemon wedge

Fill a medium sized pan up with water and place it on the burner, set at medium heat. With war water nearing the boiling point, you can then drop your lean chicken breast into the pan. Let this chicken boil for about 5 minutes before removing it from the pan. Place the chicken on a clean cutting board and let it cool down for a few moments. After cooling, start cutting the meat up with a knife until it is shredded into small pieces; dump these pieces into a medium mixing bowl.

Next, add in your fennel seeds, thyme, olive oil, and mix them together with your shredded chicken, making sure that the chicken gets well marinated with all of the ingredients. Once properly marinated like this, you can take out as much as you would like to eat and place it on a plate for consumption. As a finishing touch, slice off yourself a lemon wedge so you can sprinkle lemon juice on the shredded chicken making this paleo meal even more delicious than it already is.

Paleo Stir Fried Fajita's

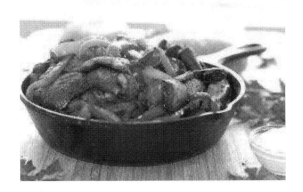

There is nothing quite like some good stir fry for your midday meal. This dish also combines some Latin flavor and spice for a much needed kick for your midday paleo routine. So mark your calendar for a day that you can enjoy yourself these deliciously paleo, stir fried fajita's!

Here are the exact ingredients:

3 pounds of beef steak

1 cup of olive oil

½ cup of crushed garlic

¼ cup of lime juice

¼ cup chili powder

¼ cup cumin

½ cup red bell pepper, chopped

½ cup yellow bell pepper, chopped

½ cup chopped onion

1 diced roma tomato

¼ cup cilantro, chopped

First put your 3 pounds of beef in a glass container. Next, take out a separate plastic container and add exactly one half of your cup of olive oil, save the rest for later, you will need it. Follow this then by adding your ½ cup of crushed garlic, ¼ cup of lime juice, ¼ cup of chili powder, and your ¼ cup of cumin. Stir these together well before pouring the entire contents of the container out on top of your beef in the glass cooking pan.

Now put your glass cooking pan in the refrigerator and let it soak up the flavor of all the ingredients for 2 hours in the fridge. Now take that other half of your olive oil that you saved and dump it into a pan and let it cook over medium heat. After this take out your glass container and dump your marinated beef steak into the pan. Next, add your onions, diced tomatoes, and peppers and let the mixture cook for a few minutes while you stir the contents. Turn off your burner and add your chopped cilantro as a finishing touch. Your Paleo Stir Fried Fajita's our now ready for consumption!

Turkey Paleo Skewers

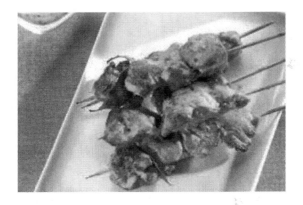

Meat on a stick? This meal is pretty straightforward and self explanatory, and even a caveman could do it! Don't worry about getting a little bit messy with this recipe, its well worth it!

Here are the exact ingredients:

5 wooden skewers

1 lean turkey breast

2 tablespoons of olive oil

2 tablespoons of chopped sage

2 tablespoons of vinegar

First take your olive oil and vinegar and mix them together well in a mixing bowl. Now set this mixture to the side and take out a clean cutting board and use it to chop up your thawed turkey breast. Add this chopped turkey breast to the mixing bowl of vinegar and oil and let it marinate in the mix for a few moments before putting a plastic covering over it and storing it in your refrigerator.

Let it stay in the fridge for a few hours, taking it out just to shift the ingredients around in the bowl every so often. After sitting in your refrigerator for a few hours, take the bowl out, and using wooden skewers, skewer the meat onto the wooden sticks. You can then cook them over an open flame such as a campfire, or over a grill making for some tasty Turkey Paleo Skewers right in the middle of your day.

Paleo Slow Cooked Chicken

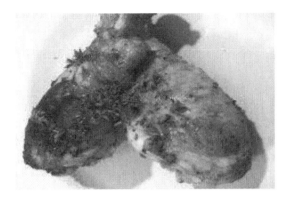

This is a hearty mid day meal right out of the Paleolithic past—that is—if the Paleolithic era had slow cookers! Because in this recipe you will find delicious chicken and juicy onions, seasoned to perfection with herbs and spices, just one slow cooked meal away from you! Just toss your chicken in the pot and get ready for a great way to kick off your midday!

Here are the exact ingredients:

2 lean chicken breasts

1 cup chopped onion

¼ cup paprika

¼ cup cayenne pepper

¼ cup black pepper

¼ cup poultry seasoning

¼ cup garlic powder

Get your slow cooker out and set it on high heat, before dropping your cup of chopped onions down to the bottom of the cooker. After you have done this, move on to blend your spices together in a medium sized mixing bowl. Add your paprika, cayenne pepper, black pepper, and poultry seasoning together and mix them well. Then take these mixed spices and pour them over your chicken breasts.

Put these now newly spiced up chicken breasts and put them right on top of the onions lining the bottom of your slow cooker. You can now put the lid on your cooker and begin the 4 to 5 hour process of cooking up this paleo mid day meal. It isn't necessary to add any water or anything like that, since your chicken breasts should have enough natural juice inside of them already. Enjoy!

Chapter 4: Supper from the Stone Age!

The last meal of the day should be able to sustain you through the rest of the night, without breaking your diet. Many of us have self control issues when we come home from a long day of work, and end up eating too much for our evening meal. In order to avoid this; simply plan it out. Take a look at these recipes and suppertime meal plans so that you can do just that!

Meaty Eggplant Meal

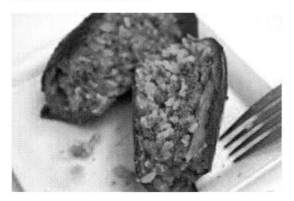

Eggplant is one of my favorite veggies, and when it is served with lean meat and fresh garlic it is even better. This meal is filling without breaking the carbohydrate bank account, and the ingredients are so simple they firmly classify as Paleolithic in their makeup. And the taste of lean hamburger meat roasted with onions and tomatoes just can't be beat! Find a place for this great recipe, at the end of your busy day.

Here are the exact ingredients:

½ pound of lean hamburger

¼ cup chopped onions

¼ cup of tomato paste

¼ cup chopped tomatoes

1 eggplant

2 cups of lettuce

The first thing you should do is cut your eggplant in half lengthwise. Put this eggplant in a baking pan and let it cook in the oven for about 10 minutes at 400 degrees Fahrenheit. While your eggplant is cooking take your hamburger and place it in a frying pan on high heat, add your cup of chopped onions and begin stirring it together vigorously as it cooks. Next, add in your tomato paste and your ¼ cup of chopped tomatoes and stir these in as well.

Now turn your burner down to low heat and let the mixture cook for another 10 minutes.

Turn off your burner and get out a large plate, spread out your lettuce on this plate and set it down on your counter. With your lettuce in place, take your cooked eggplant out of the oven and place it on top of the plate of lettuce. After you have done this you can then pour your hamburger, tomato, and onion mixture out of your frying pan and drizzle it out on top of the lettuce and eggplant. This meal is a delicious and satisfying way to have a supper that's straight out of the Stone Age.

Paleo Salmon and Chanterelle Mushroom

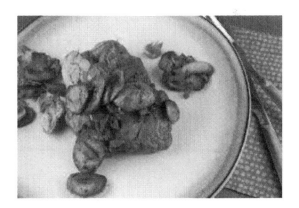

This mushroom and salmon fish dish would have been a real treat back in the Stone Age, and makes for a great supper today! Just look at this grilled fish and scrumptious mushroom combo! And nothing brings out the flavor like white wine! I hope you enjoy this Paleolithic dish, because I know I do!

Here are the exact ingredients:

3 salmon filets

1 cup of chopped chanterelle mushrooms

½ cup of olive oil

¼ cup of white wine

½ cup thyme leaves

¼ cup garlic

¼ cup butter

Set your grill to medium high, and stretch your salmon filets out on the grill. Take a marinating brush and rub some olive oil directly onto your salmon filets. Let your salmon cook. And while your salmon is cooking on the grill (or as the Australians like to call it "the Barbie"), get out a medium sized frying pan and place it on your stove with the burner set to medium.

To this pan you will add your mushrooms, garlic, butter, thyme leaves, white wine, and the rest of your olive oil. Let these cook for about 3 minutes while you stir the contents vigorously. Once cooked put your mushroom and thyme leaves mixture on a plate and add your salmon fillets to the dish. Your Stone Age Supper is now ready to eat!

Yellow Peppers, Broccoli Rabe, and Poached Egg

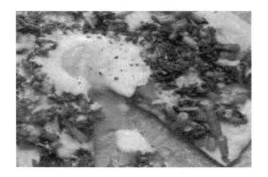

This paleo dinner dish takes the best of all natural broccoli, peppers, and eggs, and makes them into a super supper for any era! The veggies are cooked until succulently soft and the eggs just melt in your mouth! Supper is a sight to see with this Stone Age recipe!

Here are the exact ingredients:

½ cup of chopped broccoli rabe

½ cup of chopped yellow sweet peppers

¼ cup of olive oil

3 eggs

Put a pan of water on your stove and set the heat on high. Drop your half cup of chopped broccoli rabe into the pan and let it boil for about 5 minutes. After this, drain the pan of water and let your broccoli lose some of its heat. Next, add your ¼ cup of olive oil and your ½ cup of chopped yellow sweet peppers. Now, put the burner on medium heat and as you stir the mixture, let the entire contents of the pan cook for another 5 minutes. Turn the burner off and let the contents of your pan absorb the residual heat.

Setting these ingredients to the side for the moment, get out a medium sized mixing bowl and break your 3 eggs open, dropping the egg's contents inside the bowl. Cover the bowl with cling film and seal the bowl with the material. Flip the bowl upside down letting the eggs move to the surface of the film. Lift the bowl up and close the film up over the eggs, letting it seal up around them like a plastic bag. Boil the eggs while they are nestled inside this film, this will poach your paleo eggs. Now simply throw your poached eggs, yellow peppers and broccoli rabe on a plate and this Stone Age supper is ready to eat!

Shiitake Meat Loaf

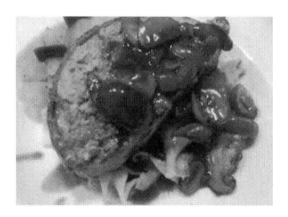

Everyone likes a little meat loaf right? Well, what about some paleo meat loaf? Cooked in rich olive oil, roasted with mushrooms and tomatoes, while being marinated by onion powder, flaxseed and red wine, this recipe is a suppertime hero. And this shiitake meat loaf blend won't disappoint!

Here are the exact ingredients:

½ cup of olive oil

¼ cup chopped shiitake mushrooms

1 cup chopped tomatoes

1 pound grass fed beef

¼ cup flaxseed

¼ cup onion powder

¼ cup red wine

2 eggs

First, preheat your oven at 400 degrees. Next put your half cup of olive oil into a frying pan and put it on a burner set on high heat. After you have done this you can then add your shiitake mushrooms and tomatoes, and let them cook for a few minutes. Now remove the pan from the burner and let it cool off for a few more minutes. You can now put the contents of the pan into a blender and blend it all together. Get out a small plastic bowl and add your 2 eggs, pound of beef, ¼ cup of flaxseed and ¼ cup of onion powder and mix them together.

Now dump this mixture into a baking pan. Use a spoon to pat down the surface of the mixture uniformly. Next, grab your pan of cooked shiitake mushrooms and tomatoes and dump them on top of the meat mixture in the pan. As a finishing touch take your ¼ cup of red wine and lightly pour it over the surface of your baking pan meat loaf mixture. Bake for about an hour, and your shiitake meat loaf is finished.

Vegetable and Beef Stew Supper

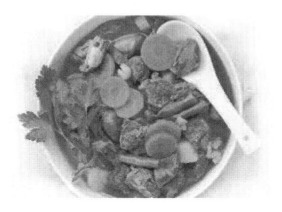

I used to love beefed stew as a kid, but as an adult the high sodium and carbs haven't always been the best thing for my diet. But the paleo version serves to fix all of that once and for all. Cooked in healthy olive oil, and roasted with paleo friendly carrots, celery, and squash, this Vegetable and Beef Stew makes for the perfect Stone Age supper!

Here are the exact ingredients:

½ cup of olive oil

1 pound of cubed chuck steak

1 cup chopped onion

½ cup of chopped garlic

1 cup chopped carrots

1 cup chopped celery

½ cup of chopped squash

1 cup chicken broth

¼ cup oregano

A dash of ground black pepper

First, add your ½ cup of olive oil to a frying pan and set your burner to medium heat. Next, add your pound of cubed steak to the pan and cook the meat until it is thoroughly brown. After you have done this, add in your chopped garlic, onion, carrots, celery and squash to the pan and stir them into the mix while they cook with the meat for another few minutes.

Now you can pour in your cup of chicken broth, bring the mixture to a boil, put on a lid, set the burner to low heat, and let the contents of the pan soak up the low heat for the next half hour. Stir regularly during this 30 minute period, and add as much black pepper as you like. Invite some friends because your vegetable and beef stew is ready for supper!

Minced Indian Curry

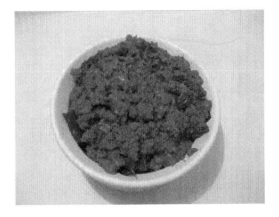

Even though curry didn't exactly exist in the Paleolithic Era, all of the ingredients that make up this batch did! So let's get ready to make some great minced Indian Curry. If Curry did exist in the Stone Age, it should have tasted like this!

Here are the exact ingredients:

1 pound of minced beef

½ cup of chopped onion

½ cup of chopped garlic

½ cup of olive oil

3 cups of chopped cabbage

1 cup of chopped eggplant

½ cup of chopped tomatoes

¼ cup of curry

To get started, go to your cutting board and begin cutting up your onion, garlic, and pound of beef. After these are properly sliced and diced throw them into a pot and turn the burner on high heat letting the contents cook for about 7 minutes. Turn the burner off and let the contents cool off for a few more minutes before dropping the ingredients into a separate container.

Now turn your burner back on high, and add your curry, chopped cabbage, chopped tomatoes, chopped eggplant and your olive oil, and start stirring the contents together.

After a few minutes of this take your separate container of the beef, onion, and garlic mixture and dump it back into the pan. Now stir everything together for a few more minutes on high heat. Turn off the burner, let the contents cool, and then serve when ready.

Paleo Barbeque Chicken

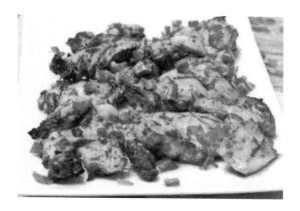

Whether it's a backyard suppertime barbeque or regular meal in the house, Paleo Barbeque Chicken won't disappoint! With lean chicken breasts cooked in healthy olive oil, and marinated with oregano, chopped garlic, and lemon juice, this Stone Age Supper is the best!

Here are the exact ingredients:

3 lean chicken breasts (A whole lot of paleo chicken!)

½ cup of olive oil

½ cup of chopped cloves of garlic

¼ cup of cumin

½ cup of oregano

¼ cup lemon juice

Mix your garlic, olive oil, paprika, cumin oregano, and lemon juice together in a small mixing bowl. With these ingredients properly mixed together take out a clean cutting board and start slicing your chicken breasts into medium sized strips. Take these strips and drop them into your mixing bowl with your other ingredients. With clean hands rub these ingredients onto your chicken breasts, let them sit in the bowl for a few more minutes, so that they can further marinate themselves.

Next, put some plastic wrap over the mixing bowl and let it sit in your refrigerator for a couple of hours, stirring it occasionally. After your marinated chicken has cooled, take out the container and take it on over to your grill. Set your grill to medium heat and place your chicken strips on top. Let these strips cook for about 15 minutes, or until they are well browned on each side. This is some of the best barbeque chicken you could ever find!

Paleo Braised River Trout

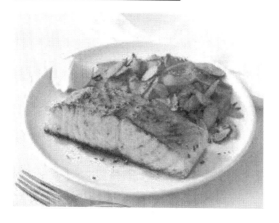

At the end of the day you need something that is both delicious and nutritious to sustain you. This Paleo Braised River Trout do just that! This type of trout is very special and is best when you catch it yourself in the wild. But if you don't have access (or time) to do all that, you can find this fish at most health food stores. Just make sure you do your homework, and you too can have your very own Paleo Braised River Trout for supper tonight!

Here are the exact ingredients:

¼ cup of olive oil

1 cup of chopped carrots

1 cup chicken broth

5 river trout fillets

A dash of black pepper

Add your ¼ cup of olive oil to a medium sized pan and set the burner to high. Next add your carrots and stir them while they cook. After you have done this you can add your cup of chicken broth and bring the whole mixture to a boil. Adjust your high heat setting to a lower one and add your fish to the pan. Sprinkle a dash of black pepper on the fish to add just the right amount of extra flavoring. Your Paleo Braised River Trout is now ready to serve and eat.

The Prehistoric Beef Tenderloin Roast

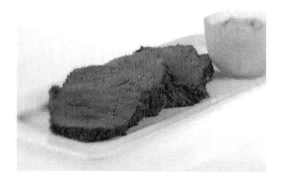

Our ancestors were eating like this before anyone knew to write about it! It was quite common for the hunter gatherers of the past to bag some wild game, roast it over the fire and then eat it with whatever other wild morsels that they found just growing in the wilderness! Just try it and you will like it! Because this fantastic dish takes grass fed beef right to the next level! With a whole pound of lean beef, cooked in olive oil marinated in flaxseed oil, chopped parsley, as well as chopped garlic and shallots, this recipe makes for a feast from the Stone Age!

Here are the exact ingredients:

1 pound of beef steak

¼ cup of olive oil

½ cup of shiitake mushrooms

¼ cup of chopped garlic

¼ cup of chopped shallots

¼ cup chopped parsley

¼ cup flaxseed oil

2 large kale leaves

To get started take your beef out of the refrigerator and let it thaw (if it isn't already) and let it sit out for about half of an hour. While your meat is thawing set your oven to about 375 degrees, to preheat. Next, add your ¼ cup of olive oil to the pan over a burner set on high. Toss in your mushrooms and vigorously stir them over the heat, and cook them for about ten minutes. After the ten minutes are up, take your mushrooms out of the pan and set them to the side.

Now put your pan back on the burner, set it to high heat, and put your pound of beef steak in the pan. In this step in the process you are just going to sear each side of the beef steak in the high heat for about 5 minutes on each side, or until brown. After doing this, take the meat out of the pan and put it in a baking pan in your already preheated oven. And while your meat is cooking, gauge the progress by inserting a meat thermometer into the steak.

Just to give you an idea of what to look for; 160 degrees signifies steak that is well done, 140 degrees is medium, 130 degrees is medium rare (that hits the spot!), and 120 degrees is rare. As anyone who has ever gone to their local steakhouse no doubt knows, everyone has a different idea of what a good steak is. Some like their steaks well done and others like them medium rare, just remember, the more undercooked your meat is the more at risk you may be for pathogens in the meat such as e coli, and salmonella.

I like a medium rare steak as much as anyone else—but it is true—the less you cook your steaks the more risk you may be taking. So going with the *happy medium*, try to cook your meat until it is medium or well done. After your meat is cooked simply add in your chopped shallots, chopped parsley, chopped garlic, and ¼ up of flaxseed oil and this Prehistoric Beef Tenderloin is ready for business!

Chapter 5: Soups, Salads, and a Few Leftovers from the Paleolithic Era

There are many great soups and salads and other leftover holdovers from the Stone Age that can be made into great paleo dishes anytime you need them. Salads in particular are a great side to any paleo meal. Paleo salads are best raw, crunchy, savory, and healthful. In the 30 Day Paleo Challenge you can really get creative with your salads. Besides the recipes given here you can feel free to add as much meat, fish, and (paleo acceptable) veggies that you want.

Much the same goes for soup too, if you would like to experiment and change up some of your soup ingredients if you like. But in the meantime take a look at some of the suggestions in this chapter as a starting place. As for your leftovers, there is no specific guideline for how to eat any leftovers from previous paleo meals and ingredients, just put them in your fridge until you can turn them into something new. This could be done in a variety of ways, and this chapter gives you some good examples. So without further adieu, here are a few of the best that the Paleolithic Era can provide!

Creamy Chicken Basil and Tomato Soup

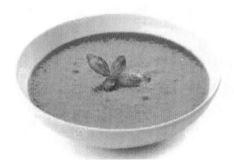

This creamy chicken treat is one of the best things you could ever eat! Just look at the ingredients! With a whole pound of quality chicken meat, cooked in the very paleo choice of coconut oil, and garnished with a wide variety of foraged foods such as sunflower seeds, onions, and even cherry tomatoes, this is a soup that you won't soon forget!

Here are the exact ingredients:

1 pound of boneless chicken thighs and breasts

½ cup of chopped onion

¼ teaspoon of coconut oil

½ cup of chopped garlic

½ cup of sunflower seeds

¼ cup of nutritional yeast

¼ cup of basil

¼ cup of avocado oil

¼ cup coconut milk

¼ cup of cold water

½ cup of chopped cherry tomatoes

To get started put your coconut oil in a big pan on medium heat, and let it warm up for a few minutes. While it's warming up add your ½ cup of chopped onions to the pan, stir your onions into your oil and then add your pound of chicken to the mix. While your chicken and onion mix are cooking in the pan. Go to your blender and add your sunflower seeds, nutrition yeast, basil and avocado oil.

Blend these ingredients together well until they are thoroughly bonded together. Pour this mixture into your pan, and allow the entire contents of the pan to cook for just a few minutes more while you thoroughly blend it all together. Now just add your ¼ cup of cold water, and ¼ cup of coconut milk, stir a few more minutes, and this Paleolithic soup is ready to serve!

Paleo Chili with Turkey

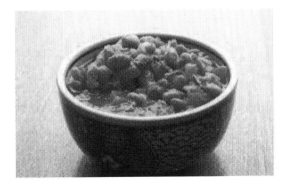

This chili may be a left over from the Paleolithic Era but it tastes just as good as any other chili I've ever had! This dish works well because it substitutes the typical ingredient in most chilies—beans—with more paleo friendly ingredients such as carrots and bell peppers. It still tastes great and you don't have to worry about the consequences of wrecking your diet (or facing the *other* consequences that beans often bring)! Ground turkey garnished with carrots, onions, bell peppers, and thyme, makes for quite a wonderful time!

Here are the exact ingredients:

½ pound of ground turkey

¼ cup of olive oil

½ cup of chopped onions

½ cup of chopped carrots

½ cup of chopped red bell peppers

½ cup of chopped yellow bell peppers

¼ cup of chopped thyme

¼ cup of ground cumin

½ cup of paprika

¼ cup of chili flakes

1 can of diced tomatoes

¼ cup of lemon juice

First, boil your ground turkey on high heat for about 15 minutes. Turn the burner off and put this pan to the side. Take out another pan and put it on medium heat. In this pan go ahead and add your bell peppers, carrots, garlic, and onions to the pan. Let these ingredients cook for just a few minutes before adding your cumin, thyme, paprika, and chili flakes to the mix. Now take a wooden spoon and vigorously whisk these ingredients together for a couple of minutes. Turn your burner to low heat, and let the ingredients simmer while you add your ground turkey to the pan. Cook the entire contents of the pan for another 10 minutes before serving.

Paleolithic Sea Bass Veggie Soup

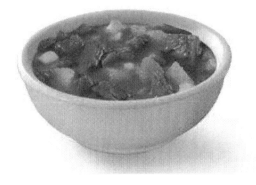

If you like fresh fish and veggies then you will love this soup! This soup is good when you want a quick nutritious meal that doesn't take a lot of work, and it goes great with a side of salad or whatever other leftovers you may have. So get your fish and veggies ready for a great bowl of soup!

Here are the exact ingredients:

¼ cup of olive oil

½ cup of chopped Sea Bass fillets

¼ cup of shiitake mushrooms

½ cup of chopped shallot

1 cup of chopped carrot

1 cup of chopped zucchini

¼ cup of chopped tomatoes

1 cup of chicken broth

First, set your oven to about 150 degrees. Next add your ¼ olive oil to a medium sized frying pan and put it on the burner of your stove. Add your chopped sea bass fillets and set your burner to high. Stir the fish as it cooks for about five minutes. After this, dump the fish into a glass baking dish; let this cook in your oven for about 15 minutes.

Now get out the rest of your olive oil and drizzle it on top of the fish, next add your chopped shallot, chopped carrot, chopped zucchini, and chopped tomatoes to the pan. Now add your cup of chicken broth, pouring it evenly over the top of the ingredients. Let this cook for a few more minutes and this Paleolithic soup is ready to go!

Paleo Salmon Caesar Salad

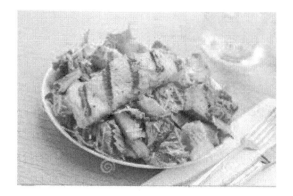

Fresh Caesar salad is delicious and this paleo blend is even better! The Omega 3s in particular that are found in this dish make for a great part of a paleo diet. A good dose of Omega 3 can help decrease your risk for cardiovascular disease, prevent the development of arthritis and even cure depression, all great reasons to have a goof Caesar salad!

Here are the exact ingredients:

3 salmon fillets

¼ cup of olive oil

1 head of chopped romaine lettuce

½ cup of chopped onion

¼ cup of flaxseed oil

¼ cup of crushed garlic

¼ cup of mustard seed

¼ cup of lemon juice

A dash of black pepper

Take a cooking brush and use it to drench your salmon fillets with your olive oil. Put them into a baking pan and broil in the oven for about 10 minutes. After which take the salmon out and set it aside. Now take out a mixing bowl, add your lettuce and chopped onion, and mix in your flaxseed oil, mustard seed, garlic, and lemon juice. Once you have stirred these together, put your salmon on top of it and your Paleo Salmon Caesar Salad.

Chicken Zoodle Soup

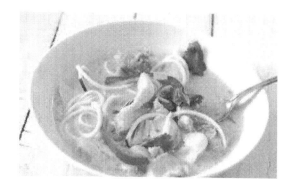

We all love Chicken Noodle soup, especially when we are suffering from a bad cold, or just plain need a comfort food. But for the Paleo diet however, the original Chicken Noodle soup recipe is loaded with unhealthy carbohydrates not conducive for a paleo diet. Fortunately, with a little bit of Stone Age engineering, those noodles can be replaced with zoodles! Yes, zoodles; zucchini sliced into long noodles! They have just about the same consistency of pasta without all those pesky carbs! And they taste great in soup, and offer a tasty respite for your 30 Day Paleo Challenge!

Here are the exact ingredients:

1 medium sized Zucchini

1 cup of chicken stock

1 lean chicken breast

2 cups of water

In order to create your chicken zoodle soup you don't need much, just a zucchini, chicken stock, a chicken breast, and some water. First, boil your chicken breast in a pan for about 10 minutes on high heat. Let the chicken cool before taking it out of the pan, and shredding the chicken into small pieces, set this to the side for now in a separate container.

Go back to your pan and add your cup of chicken stock and your 2 cups of water, briefly stir contents together and turn your burner back on, set to medium heat. While the soup mixture is heating up go to your cutting board, take out your medium zucchini and start slicing with a vegetable peeler as thin as you can, lengthwise. Add these noodles to the cooking soup and stir for a few minutes as they simmer in the pan. Finally, add your shredded chicken to the pan, cook for about five additional minutes and turn the burner off. This chicken zoodle soup is on!

Chicken Salad and Walnuts

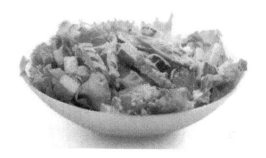

This salad will fill you up and not bust your paleo dietary budget! All you need is one lean chicken breast, some arugula leaves, a bit of seasoning and some walnuts and your chicken salad is complete!

Here are the exact ingredients:

1 lean chicken breast

¼ cup of Cajun chicken seasoning

¼ cup of chopped walnuts

2 cups of arugula leaves

1 green apple, sliced and diced

¼ cup of lemon juice

¼ cup of honey

¼ cup of olive oil

¼ cup of vinegar

Set your oven to 400 degrees. Get out an oven tray and place some baking safe paper down at the bottom of it. Next, get out your cutting board and cut up your chicken breast into finely chopped pieces. Put your freshly chopped chicken into a plastic bowl, from here; begin drizzling your ¼ cup of Cajun chicken seasoning onto your chopped chicken. After you have done this put your chicken pieces and put them on your oven tray, and place the tray into the oven. Let's these cook for at least 10 minutes.

With your chicken in the oven, now you can turn to the preparation of the rest of your ingredients. First, put your ¼ cup of chopped walnuts, put them in a pan, and set the burner to high. Now just let these nuts roast until they turn brown, occasionally stirring them. After this, take out your arugula leaves, your sliced and diced apples, your ¼ cup of honey, ¼ cup of lemon juice, ¼ cup of olive oil, and your ¼ cup of vinegar and put them in a small mixing bowl. Stir the contents of your bowl together before dumping the contents onto a large plate; this will constitute the salad of your *chicken salad*. Just take your chopped chicken out of the oven and put it right on top of this paleo-terrific plate of salad!

The Duck Burger Leftover

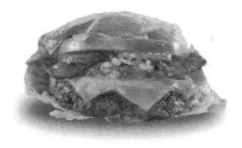

If you dined on a scrumptious bit of roasted duck the night before and still have plenty left over the next day, you can always turn the remnants into a delicious duck burger! This is a fine paleo delicacy! Duck has a very savory taste and once you experience it, you may never want to go back to regular hamburgers ever again! That's quite an accomplishment from food that was merely a *leftover*!

Here are the exact ingredients:

1 pound of leftover duck

¼ cup of chopped rosemary

¼ cup of chopped garlic

¼ cup of chopped onions

½ cup chopped tomatoes

1 head of butter lettuce

Dash of pepper

2 eggs

Chop up your leftover duck (if it isn't already) into small little pieces. Now put this meat in a grinder to further grind it up, and then deposit the ground meat into a medium sized mixing bowl. Next, add your eggs, rosemary, and chopped garlic to the meat and stir these ingredients together well, before taking your bare (clean!) hands and shaping the ground duck into hamburger styled patties. Just smooth and mold them together until your ground duck meat somewhat resembles the shape of a hamburger!

Place these patties on a large plate and season however you wish (I usually sprinkle mine with a liberal amount of pepper!) Now one by one, add these duck patties to the frying pan and let them cook for about 15 minutes on each side. Add your chopped tomatoes and onions while the meat is cooking. Once your duck burger patties have finished cooking just put them in between your leaves of lettuce and this Leftover Duck Burger is ready for you to take a bite!

Paleo Posole Soup

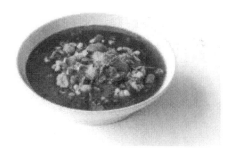

This thick and tasty soup is a variation of the classic pork posole, but instead of carb rich ingredients such as hominy grits, this paleo version of pasole soup uses a delicious blend of refined squash. This dish is as tasty as it is hearty and can serve up to 3 people, making it a great dish for you and two of your fellow paleo diet guests. Otherwise your pasole remnants will make for some great leftovers later on. Don't forget to try out this recipe during your 30 Day Paleo Challenge!

Here are the exact ingredients:

1 pound of pork shoulder

½ cup of chopped onion

½ cup of garlic

½ cup of cumin

¼ cup of oregano

¼ cup of red pepper flakes

¼ cup of olive oil

¼ cup of cilantro

2 cups of water

1 cup of chopped squash

First put your pork shoulder in a medium sized pot and add your 2 cups of water, ½ cup of chopped onion, ½ cup of garlic, ½ cup of cumin, ¼ cup of oregano, and ¼ cup of red pepper flakes. Let this mixture boil, stir briefly, and then cover the pot. Now take your burner down to a low heat setting and allow your pot to simmer for a little over an hour. After your hour as passed, turn the burner off and pour the contents of the pot into a large bowl. Now place your pot back on the burner and set to medium heat, reheating the oily remnants in the pot.

Next, add your chopped squash to the pot and allow these veggies to cook in the oil for about 7 minutes, stirring them so that they become evenly brown on all sides. Now you can put your meat and other ingredients back into the pan. Set your burner back on low heat and let the entire mixture slow cook for about an hour and a half. After an hour and a half, your meat and veggies should be extremely juicy and tender. Finnish things off by adding your cilantro on top and you are done!

Leftover Hash

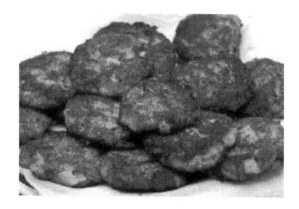

Just because it's leftover doesn't mean it's not going to be good! Take this leftover hash as a prime example! All you got to do is take a little bit of beef and mix up with some sweet potato, chopped onions, and tomato sauce and you are in for a delicious leftover from the Paleolithic Era!

Here are the exact ingredients:

1 cup chopped sweet potato

½ cup of chopped onion

¼ pound of beef or hamburger leftovers

½ cup tomato sauce

¼ cup of coconut oil

Get started on the main component of your leftover hash first; the sweet potato. Chop this sweet potato up into small pieces. Next, chop up your onion, until you have about half a cup. After that, place a large sauce pan on medium heat and add your coconut oil to the pan. Let this heat up for about 30 seconds before adding your sweet potatoes, onions, tomato sauce and of course, your ¼ of a pound of leftover beef or hamburger. Stir this mixture together, let it cook for about 5 minutes, and these leftovers from the Stone Age are complete!

Chapter 6: A few Good Paleo Desserts and Beverages

Even a caveman needs a good dessert every now and then! Thankfully there are several alterations you can make to classic dessert staples. These alterations, allow for the creation of great desserts and beverages without deviating from the paleo routine. The guidelines for paleo desserts are pretty basic; just avoid grains and refined sugar and focus instead on maximizing what you can get from nuts, spices, dried fruits, and veggies. You can shred some carrots for example, and make some pretty mean paleo carrot cake. Its simple food ideas like this that help make the 30 Day Paleo Challenge so sustainable.

Baked Paleo Apple Desert

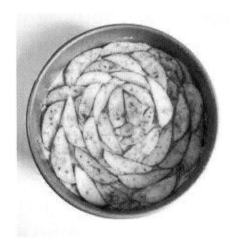

As good as an old fashioned apple pie, these Baked Paleo Apples are just as tasty even without the heavily processed gluten filled crust of typical apple based deserts. So forget all about that apple pie and give this paleo dessert recipe a try!

Here are the exact ingredients:

¼ cup of raisins

¼ cup raw walnuts

¼ cup cinnamon

1 cup of chopped apples

½ cup of water

First, set your oven to 400 degrees. Next, take your ¼ cup of raisins, ¼ cup of walnuts, ¼ cup of cinnamon, and mix them together in a medium sized mixing bowl. Now transfer these ingredients to a glass baking pan, and add your cup of chopped apples to the mix as well. Add your ½ cup of water and thoroughly mix your ingredients together. Put this mixture in the oven and let it cook for about a half hour. After which your baked paleo apple dessert is ready to serve.

Caveman Crème and Strawberries

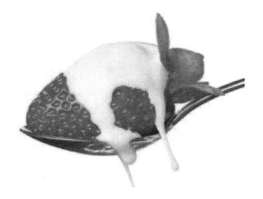

This dessert is a classic with a paleo twist. Fresh strawberries served without the excess of sweet sugary additives that accompany them. This dish takes out those non paleo elements and transforms it into something truly great! If you need a pick me up during your 30 Day Paleo Challenge, give this Caveman Crème and Strawberries recipe a look over!

Here are the exact ingredients:

2 cups strawberries, sliced

¼ cup of vanilla extract

¼ cup of coconut milk

This recipe requires some special preparation so you are going to have to put a whisk and a copper bowl up inside your freezer in order to chill them for about 25 minutes. Now take out another bowl and add your vanilla extract and strawberries, stir these together before covering them and putting them in the fridge.

Next, add your coconut milk to the other bowl that you left in the refrigerator for 25 minutes, and then take your whisk and use it to stir the coconut milk, letting it thicken. This is all you have to do to thicken your crème. Now take your other bowl and dump your strawberries and vanilla into your thickened crème mixture. Your Caveman Crème and Strawberries are now ready to eat.

Paleo Banana Bonanza

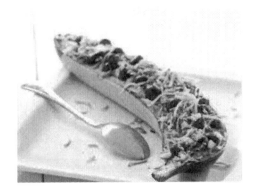

Banana's are a fruit to be reckoned with on the paleo diet. One of the great things about bananas is the fact that they are so versatile. And with the help of a few key ingredients—as shown in this recipe—you can really make a dessert that everyone will like. Its sweet and its crunchy, and its altogether delicious. You don't even have to be a caveman to enjoy this Paleo Banana Bonanza.

Here are the exact ingredients:

2 large, ripened bananas

¼ of a cup of vanilla extract

¼ cup of ginger

¼ cup of allspice

¼ cup of pecans

This dessert really takes the cake (no pun intended). This simple banana recipe makes for a great paleo treat loaded with potassium! To get started, cut your bananas vertically and then put them in a small container. Next, put the bananas face down on a piece of paper wax, before putting them in the freezer and letting them cool down for about half an hour. After this take the bananas out and drizzle your ginger, allspice, pecans, and nutmeg on top of the bananas. Now you can truly have yourself a Paleo Banana Bonanza!

Mango Margarita

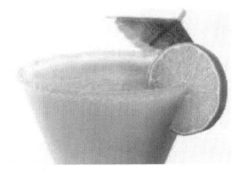

Smooth, cool, and refreshing! This Mango Margarita mix bypasses the corn syrup of other processed sweet drinks, and gives you an even better paleo alternative! There is simply nothing better after a hot summer day than a nice cool round of Mango Margaritas!

Here are the exact ingredients:

1 cup of water

1 cup of mango cubes

½ cup of lime juice

This recipe is about as straight forward as it gets, simply take your cup of water, mango cubes, and lime juice and put them in a blender. Blend these ingredients together, pour in a glass, and get ready to drink up.

Chapter 7: Tips for Making Paleo Work; 30 Days and Beyond

Starting an ambitious plan such as the 30 Day Paleo Challenge will no doubt, leave you with some questions. In this chapter we seek to answer some of the most frequent of them. Here they are in no particular order; tips for making paleo work!

Why Organic Veggies and Grass Fed Meat?

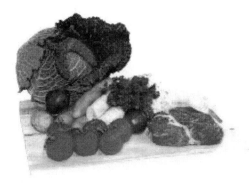

The simplest answer to this is because organic veggies and grass fed meat are in their most natural (most Paleolithic) state. To go into a bit further detail however, the main problem with processed veggies and meat is all of the additives and treatments that they were subjected to before they got put on your plate. All of the growth hormones, pesticides, and chemicals that regular store bought food tends to have, cause quite a bit of unhealthy inflammation in the body, creating a very *un-paleo* over all condition for our health.

But naturally grown organic veggies and grass fed animals are free from these man mad manipulations and are in a much more natural and balanced state, just like our Paleolithic, hunter gatherer, forefathers intended. You will be amazed by the diversity of textures, tastes, and colors of the veggies you will use during your 30 Day Paleo Challenge, but it is the sheer nutritional value of these veggies that will stand out the most.

The same thing can be said for grass fed meat as well, because besides animals hunted and snatched up directly from the wild, grass fed, free ranging domestic animals produce the healthiest meat you could ever eat. The same goes for the eggs that these animals produce, creating much healthier and more nutritious egg yolk for your paleo diet. These benefits can be directly attributed to the environment that these animals are raised in.

The fact that they are allowed to roam around freely and eat their own grass fed food naturally by grazing around, makes the animal itself much healthier. So much so, that they yield leaner meat full of beneficial omega 3 fatty acids (this is the good fat) and much less of the unhealthy saturated fat that grain fed farm animals are afflicted with. You can actually tell the difference between grass fed meat and grain fed meat simply by looking at it. Just think about the appearance of your typical grocery store bought bacon. You probably see a lot of reddish and white hues in the meat right?

The white parts that you see in this bacon are accumulations of saturated fat, developed from the lifetime of unhealthy, mass produced feed grain that this poor animal spent eating. If you were to buy bacon that came from a grass fed animal however, instead of white fat deposits, you would see the distinctive bright orange colorings indicative of an animal that spent its life consuming healthy and natural grass.

It is actually the vitamin beta-carotene that gives grass fed fat its color. This same vitamin known for its presence in carrots, is also present in the grass that grass fed animals consume, giving their fat deposits a bright orange hue. Beta-carotene is good for humans too, that's why we can benefit so much by eating grass fed meat that is loaded with it.

If you don't have a local butcher to obtain grass fed meat from, many local health food stores have begun to specialize in the practice, be sure to ask around for this important aspect of the paleo diet. Grass fed beef and organic veggies are not something that you can substitute with something else, you have to have the real thing. So take your time, and make sure you get this right.

What's up with Fat?

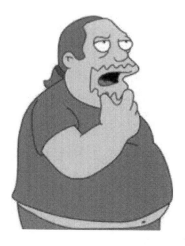

All of your life you have probably been told that fat is bad, and sought to avoid it as much as you could. That's what low fat diets are all about right? But contrary to conventional wisdom and popular opinion, some fats are actually good for you; it just depends on what kind of fat it is. Fat helps our body replenish its energy and it is fat that actually gives us that fulfilling "full" feeling after a meal.

Fats also help you to absorb nutrients. That's why cutting all fat from your diet can make you so unhealthy. Without any fat, your body struggles to even nourish itself. But having that said, it depends on the kinds of fats you are consuming as mentioned earlier in this chapter, the fat from grass fed meat is beneficial but the fat from grain fed animals is not. But fat from meat is not the only area you should be concerned with.

In addition to meat fats, for paleo, plant based fats are a must. Fats from coconut oil, nuts, and avocados for example, can be an amazing help and integral part of the paleo diet. These fats not only help you shed pounds, they are also good for your hair and skin! A diet of *good fat* will help the sheen and shimmer of your hair and nails. But fats from vegetable oil or any other highly processed material will only wreck your diet. You can most definitely use some fat during the 30 Day Paleo Challenge; it just has to be the right kind!

What's a Good Caloric Intake on Paleo?

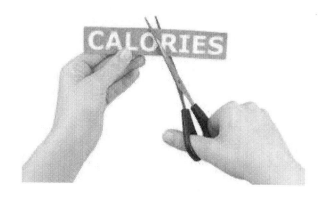

Unlike other diets such as the "Atkins Diet", which have you counting an exact number of carbs. The Paleo diet—in this sense—is not a carb counting diet plan. Rather than focusing on the exact quantity of carbs you consume, the paleo diet is much more concerned with the *quality* of carbs that you take into your body. If you find yourself still hungry after your main meal of calories, don't deprive yourself just to maintain a trivial calorie count, go ahead and eat! Just make sure that you are eating quality food, such as meat high in protein, or even foods high in plant based fat like nuts and coconut oil. This is the fuel that your 30 Day Paleo Challenge runs on!

Where can I find Free Range Poultry?

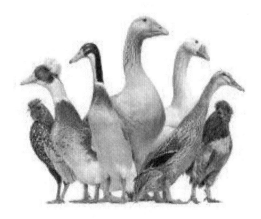

Free range chickens and other poultry are the best, but where can you find them? This is a number one question for many who embark upon the 30 Day Paleo Challenge. Free ranging birds that live on a natural diet of bugs and grass are the best option for our health, and worth the effort of locating them.

Start off your search by going to www.eatwild.com. This site holds one of the best search engines when it comes to finding a local supplier of free ranger poultry. Just type in your location and the kind of poultry you are looking for (chicken, turkey, duck, goose, pheasant, quail; etcetera). You can also contact "Games International" a nation wide distributor of wild game in order to obtain free range poultry as well. You can contact them at:

Game Sales International

P.O. Box 7719

Loveland, CO 80537

(800) 729-2090

Another option for you could be a local farmer's market, most towns have them; you just have to find them. These are all great places to find free range poultry. Once you find a resource that works with you, just stick with it, and you will be able to greatly streamline the whole process of your 30 Day Paleo Challenge.

Does Snacking Wreck the Paleo Diet?

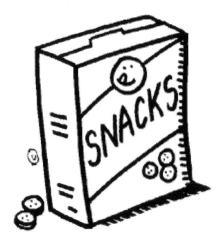

Much of the craving we feel for snacks, happens as a side effect of eating overly processed food. Many who start the paleo diet are amazed at just how much these cravings subside once their paleo diet begins. But most of these cravings will diminish after your system gets used to burning the *more quality* fat intake that the paleo diet runs on, helping to balance your blood sugar and reduce the snacking habit. But having that said, if you do still feel the urge to snack, among the best options to choose from would be grass fed beef, nuts or even seeds. So yes, feel free to have a snack!

What about Coffee and Alcohol?

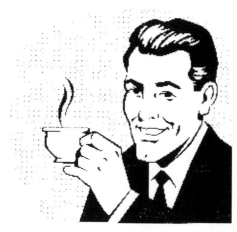

There is no way to sugar coat this one; coffee and alcohol can prove harmful, sometimes even fatal to your efforts of making the 30 Day Paleo Challenge work. You have to be very careful if you choose to continue their consumption. Beer of course, is heavy in harmful carbohydrates and it's so called "empty calories" have next to no nutritional value for your body. Beer is one of the worst of the alcoholic offenders; vodka on the other hand isn't all that bad. Clear alcohol just doesn't have the carb and caloric woes of other alcoholic beverages.

This is the typical paleo stance on alcohol, but when it comes to coffee the best thing you could possibly do is drink it black. Because black coffee devoid of any cream, sugar, or sweetener; is in its most natural, most Paleolithic state. Even so, try to keep your coffee levels down to a minimum of just 1 or 2 cups a day. This may disappoint some of you Starbucks fans out there, but your body could probably use a break from the caffeine as well, so at least for the duration of your 30 Day Paleo Challenge, try to keep it to a minimum.

What Kinds of Changes Should I Expect?

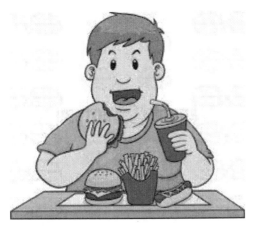

Any change in life can be difficult, and this is especially true with our diets. We get so used to eating certain foods, when those foods are taken away we not only feel deprived, we actually go into withdrawal. Recent studies have even shown that carb heavy foods such as pasta and junk food such as potato chips are so addictive that the first few days of their removal from your diet could cause headaches and stomach pain! But despite such difficulties by the end of your 30 Day Paleo challenge these problems will be quite mitigated, and you will feel better than ever.

Exactly How Much Protein Should I Consume on

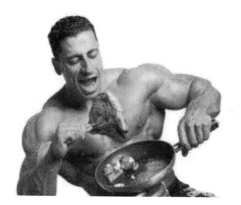

Paleo?

The amount of protein that you should consume actually hinges upon your own personal bodyweight. Most should aim for about 1 gram of protein per pound. Based on your own weight you can take this formula and use it for your own calculations. One interesting thing about the protein in paleo based food, is that it isn't quite as readily processed by the body as store processed food. This means that you have to actually work a little bit harder to digest it. It might sound a bit odd, but if you wish to consume better protein on the paleo diet, you need to *really chew* your food!

People don't much realize or think about it, but the mouth itself is an important digestive organ and contains several important enzymes that jumpstart the digestive process as soon as you start chewing. Having that said; protein from paleo based food are much better utilized when you actually take the time to chew your food well and allow those enzymes to do their job. So remember when your mom said to "slow down an chew your food"? Well, guess what; she was right!

How Would Autoimmune Deficiencies Affect Paleo?

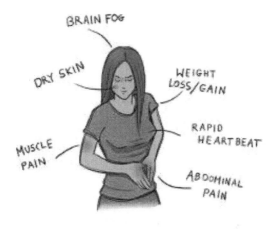

This is a valid question and concern. If you have an autoimmune disease you should probably avoid eggs, butter, and potatoes. Also avoid seeds and nuts, and you might even have to limit your intake of fruit. Because these are all known to work as gut irritants, and almost all autoimmune diseases are caused by a poor gut health to begin with. Most people are not aware of this, but right next to cancer and heart disease, autoimmune diseases afflict more people than any other disease.

In the United States alone, autoimmune diseases affect an estimated 15 million people at any given time. Some of the most common autoimmune diseases that people suffer from are rheumatoid arthritis, multiple sclerosis, and of course, the ever frequent, ulcerative colitis. But basically, an auto immune disease can be defined as any condition in which the body's own immune system has lost its capacity to tell the difference between healthy tissue cells and outside agents.

This confused condition results in the body's immune system "automatically" attacking your own healthy cell structure, leading to the painful symptoms of this disease. In ulcerative colitis for example, it is this excessive response from the immune system that attacks certain protein deposits in the colon, causing major dysfunction in the body. If you have an autoimmune disease, in order to cure this problem you need to take some drastic action—at least for the first 30 days—so that you can get rid of these kinds of symptoms.

During the first month of your paleo diet you need to make sure that your kitchen is the focal point of your experience. Everything in your diet should begin and end in the kitchen. By making sure that your kitchen only houses food that is good for you, you can make sure that you maintain your freedom from disease and suffering, including suffering from autoimmune deficiencies.

In answer to the question, if tweaked appropriately, the paleo diet can actually be very beneficial for those that suffer from autoimmune disease. Paleo is helpful because the diet lacks grains, especially lectin and saponin based grains. Just by cutting these from your diet, you can head off much of the autoimmune disease problem at the pass. This is preventative medicine at its finest.

Another reason that paleo can be helpful is the fact that it removes milk consumption (at least processed milk), from the diet. Since processed dairy products have been known to cause many instances of autoimmune disorders such as type 1 diabetes, and other afflictions, its removal from the diet can have tremendous benefit. So if you have an autoimmune disease, pay special attention during your 30 Day Paleo Challenge and adjust your diet accordingly.

Conclusion: It Doesn't Take a Paleontologist

Congratulations! For thirty days you have went back to your Paleolithic roots, reintroducing to your body the joys of grass fed, natural meat, non-contaminated veggies, and purely grown seeds, nuts, and fruit. You did all of this while avoiding McDonalds, bypassing the potato chips, and leaving every vestige of processed food behind. But now the question needs to be asked; what should you do at the end of your 30 Day Paleo Challenge?

First of all, I would like to suggest; celebrate! Reward yourself for a job well done! Also take note of the areas in which you saw the most improvements and the place in which you felt the strongest challenges. With this honest review of your progress you can then better refine the future lifestyle choices that you are going to want to make as you take the Paleo Challenge 30 days and beyond! It doesn't take a Paleontologist to know that you are on the brink of being the healthiest you have ever been! The results speak for themselves! Thank you for reading!